JUICING FOR WEIGHT LOSS

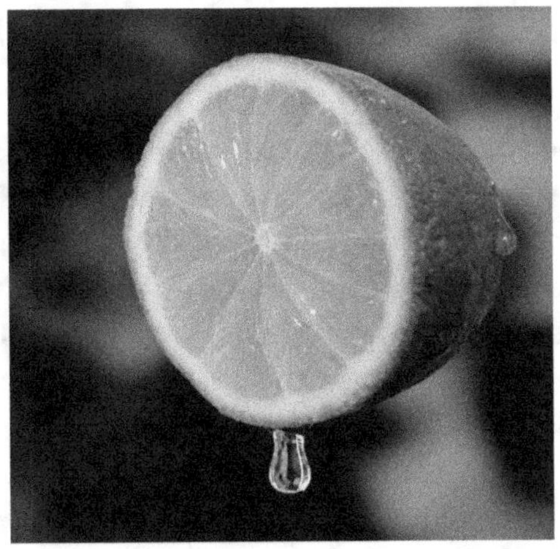

Easy Steps To A Healthier Slimmer You

BY

Kristi Wallace

TABLE OF CONTENTS

INTRODUCTION

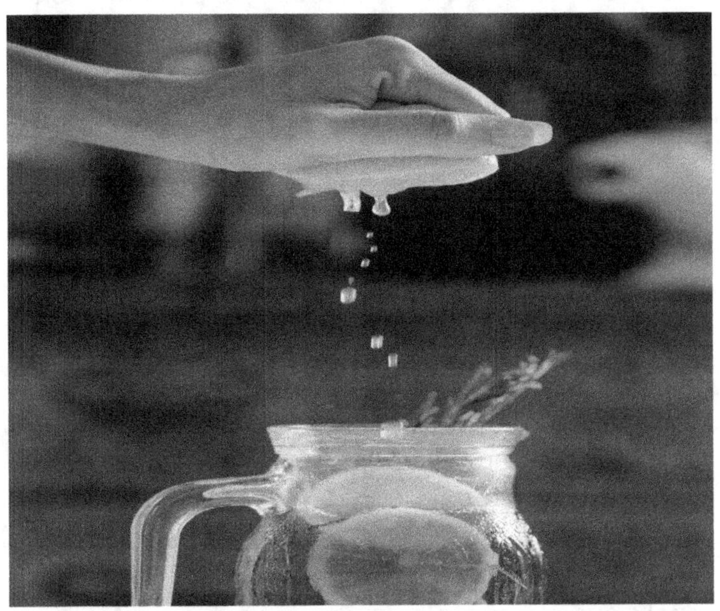

Welcome to "Juicing for Weight Loss," a comprehensive guide designed to help you harness the power of fresh fruits and vegetables to achieve your weight loss goals. In today's fast-paced world, finding a sustainable and healthy way to lose weight can be challenging. Fad diets and quick fixes often fail to deliver long-term results, leaving many feeling frustrated and defeated. This book offers a natural, nutrient-rich solution that not only supports weight loss but also promotes overall well-being.

Juicing is more than just a trend; it's a lifestyle choice that can transform your relationship with food and your body. By extracting juice from fresh produce, you can enjoy a delicious, low-calorie beverage that is packed with essential vitamins, minerals, and antioxidants. These nutrients play a crucial role in boosting metabolism, improving digestion, and providing the energy needed to stay active and healthy.

In this book, you will find a variety of juicing recipes tailored to support weight loss, detoxification, and overall health. We'll explore the science behind juicing, the benefits of different fruits and vegetables, and practical tips for incorporating juicing into your daily routine. Whether you are a juicing novice or an experienced enthusiast, this guide will provide you with valuable insights and delicious recipes to help you on your weight loss journey.

Join me as we delve into the vibrant world of juicing, where each glass is a step towards a healthier, happier you. Let's embark on this journey together, unlocking the potential of natural, wholesome ingredients to achieve lasting weight loss and a revitalized life.

The Benefits of Juicing

1. Increased Nutrient Intake

- **Vitamins and Minerals:** Juicing allows you to consume a wide variety of fruits and vegetables, ensuring a rich intake of essential vitamins and minerals.

- **Antioxidants:** Juices are packed with antioxidants, which help combat oxidative stress and reduce the risk of chronic diseases.

- **Phytochemicals:** These natural compounds found in plants have numerous health benefits, including anti-inflammatory and immune-boosting properties.

2. Improved Digestion and Detoxification.

- **Simpler Absorption:** The breakdown of fruit and vegetable cell walls while juicing facilitates your body's absorption of nutrients.

- **Digestive Health**: The enzymes in fresh juice can aid in digestion and support a healthy gut.

- **Detoxification**: Juices help flush out toxins from your body, promoting overall detoxification and improved liver function.

3. Weight Loss Support

- **Low-Calorie Intake**: Juices are typically low in calories, which can help reduce overall calorie consumption.

- **Appetite Control**: Drinking juice can help control cravings and reduce the temptation to snack on unhealthy foods.

- **Boosted Metabolism**: Certain ingredients in juices, such as ginger and cayenne pepper, can boost your metabolism and enhance fat burning.

4. Enhanced Energy Levels

- **Quick Nutrient Delivery**: Juices provide a quick source of energy due to their high nutrient density and rapid absorption.

- **Reduced Fatigue**: Consuming fresh juice can combat fatigue and increase overall vitality, helping you stay active and energetic.

5. Better Skin Health

- **Hydration:** Juices are hydrating, which is essential for maintaining healthy skin.

- **Skin-Nourishing Nutrients**: Vitamins and antioxidants found in juices, such as vitamin C and beta-carotene, contribute to clearer, more radiant skin.

6. Improved Immune Function

- **Immune-Boosting Ingredients**: Ingredients like citrus fruits, leafy greens, and berries are rich in vitamin C and other immune-boosting compounds.

- **Infection Resistance**: Regular consumption of nutrient-rich juices can strengthen your immune system, making you less susceptible to infections.

7. Convenience and Variety

- **Easy Preparation:** Juicing is a quick and convenient way to consume a variety of fruits and vegetables, especially for those with a busy lifestyle.

- **Taste and Enjoyment**: Juicing allows for creative combinations, making it easy to enjoy the taste and health benefits of different produce.

8. Mental Clarity and Focus

- **Brain Health:** The nutrients in fresh juice, such as folate and antioxidants, support brain health and improve cognitive function.

- **Mood Enhancement:** Regular consumption of nutrient-dense juices can positively impact your mood and reduce stress levels.

9. Supports Heart Health

- **Cholesterol Management:** Certain fruits and vegetables in juices, such as beets and pomegranates, can help lower cholesterol levels.

- **Blood Pressure Regulation:** Juices rich in potassium, like those from leafy greens and citrus fruits, help regulate blood pressure and promote cardiovascular health.

These benefits make juicing a powerful addition to a healthy lifestyle, particularly for those aiming for weight loss and overall wellness.

How Juicing Aids Weight Loss

1. Low-Calorie Intake

- **Caloric Deficit:** Juicing can help create a caloric deficit, which is essential for weight loss. Fresh juices are typically low in calories but high in nutrients, allowing you to consume fewer calories while still getting essential vitamins and minerals.

- **Reduced Caloric Density**: Replacing high-calorie snacks or meals with low-calorie juices can significantly reduce overall daily calorie intake.

2. Nutrient Density

- **High Nutrient Content**: Juices made from fresh fruits and vegetables are packed with essential nutrients such as vitamins, minerals, and antioxidants, which support overall health and can help prevent nutrient deficiencies during weight loss.

- **Improved Satiety:** Nutrient-dense juices can help you feel full and satisfied, reducing the temptation to overeat or snack on unhealthy foods.

3. Boosted Metabolism

- **Thermogenic Ingredients**: Certain ingredients commonly used in juicing, such as ginger, cayenne pepper, and green tea, have thermogenic properties that can boost your metabolism and increase the rate at which your body burns calories.

- **Enhanced Fat Burning**: Ingredients like lemon, grapefruit, and green vegetables can help enhance fat oxidation and promote the breakdown of stored fat.

4. Appetite Control

- **Fiber Content**: While juicing typically removes some fiber, adding ingredients like chia seeds or using a blender instead of a juicer can retain fiber, helping to control appetite by promoting a feeling of fullness.

- **Hormonal Regulation:** Some juices can help regulate hunger hormones, such as ghrelin and leptin, aiding in better appetite control and reduced cravings.

5. Detoxification and Digestion

- **Liver Support:** Juices rich in detoxifying ingredients like beets, cilantro, and dandelion greens support liver function, helping your body eliminate toxins more efficiently and potentially aiding in weight loss.

- **Improved Digestion:** Enzymes in fresh juice can improve digestion and nutrient absorption, promoting a healthier digestive tract which is crucial for effective weight management.

6. Hydration

- **Increased Water Intake:** Juices contribute to your daily water intake, ensuring you stay hydrated. Proper hydration is essential for metabolism and can help reduce water retention and bloating.

- **Enhanced Cellular Function:** Well-hydrated cells function more efficiently, supporting overall metabolic processes and energy expenditure.

7. Increased Energy Levels

- **Immediate Energy Boost:** The natural sugars and nutrients in fresh juice provide a quick source of energy, helping to combat fatigue and maintain physical activity levels, which are important for burning calories.

- **Sustained Energy**: Consistent consumption of nutrient-rich juices can lead to sustained energy levels throughout the day, supporting an active lifestyle that promotes weight loss.

8. Meal Replacement and Portion Control

- **Convenient Meal Replacements**: Juices can be used as convenient meal replacements, especially for breakfast or lunch, helping to control portion sizes and reduce overall calorie intake.

- **Structured Eating Patterns:** Incorporating juicing into your daily routine can help establish more structured eating patterns, reducing the likelihood of overeating.

9. Reduced Cravings for Unhealthy Foods

- **Satisfying Sweet Tooth:** Fruit-based juices can satisfy sweet cravings in a healthy way, reducing the temptation to indulge in sugary snacks and desserts.

- **Increased Vegetable Intake**: Juicing can make it easier to consume vegetables that you might not otherwise include in your diet, providing essential nutrients that help curb cravings for less healthy foods.

10.   Psychological Benefits

- **Mindful Eating**: Juicing encourages mindfulness about what you consume, fostering a greater awareness of healthy eating habits.

- **Positive Reinforcement**: Seeing and feeling the positive effects of juicing on your body can provide motivation and reinforce your commitment to a healthy lifestyle and weight loss goals.

By incorporating juicing into your diet, you can leverage these benefits to support and enhance your weight loss efforts, making it a sustainable and enjoyable part of your health and wellness journey.

CHAPTER ONE

The basics of Juicing

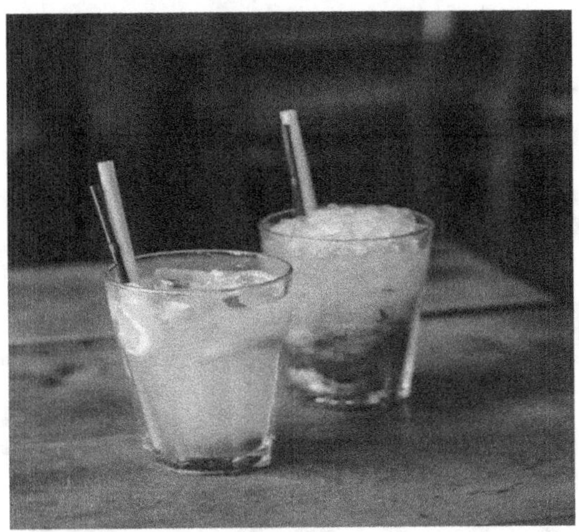

What is juicing?

Juicing is a process where you extract the juice from fresh raw fruits and vegetables, separating the pulp and fiber from the liquid.The juice of fruits or vegetables is rich in vitamins, minerals, and antioxidants.

Juicing facilitates the body's ability to absorb and process huge amounts of nutrients. You can get more vitamins, minerals, and antioxidants from a single glass of fresh juice than you could possibly consume in a single meal.

TYPES OF JUICER

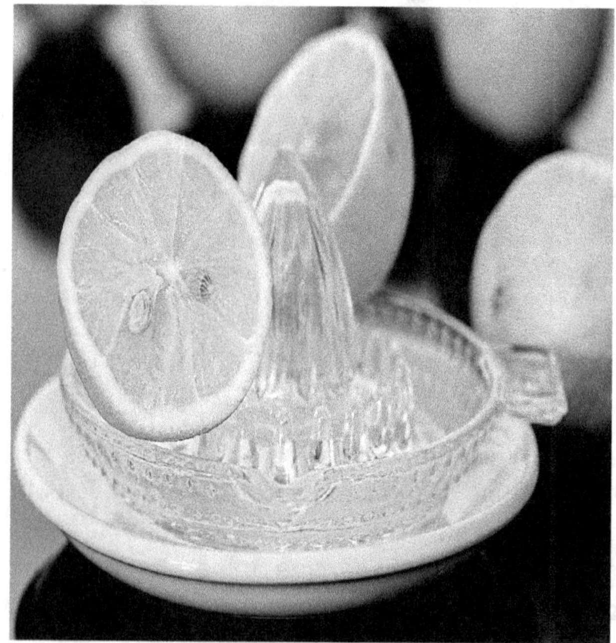

Understanding the different types of juicers available can help you choose the right one for your needs:

Centrifugal Juicers:

- **How They Work:** Use a high-speed spinning blade to chop up fruits and vegetables, then separate the juice from the pulp through centrifugal force.

- **Pros:** Fast, affordable, and easy to use.
- **Cons:** Can be noisy, less efficient at juicing leafy greens, and the juice may have a shorter shelf life due to oxidation.

1. Masticating Juicers:

- **How They Work:** Use a slow, grinding mechanism to crush fruits and vegetables, extracting juice by pressing them through a mesh screen.

- **Pros:** More efficient at juicing leafy greens, produce higher juice yield, and the juice has a longer shelf life.
- **Cons:** Slower and more expensive than centrifugal juicers.

2. Twin-Gear Juicers:

- **How They Work:** Use two interlocking gears to crush and press fruits and vegetables.

- **Pros:** Highly efficient at extracting juice, great for leafy greens, nuts, and wheatgrass, and produce high-quality juice with minimal oxidation.
- **Cons:** Expensive, large, and typically more complex to clean.

3. Citrus Juicers:

- **How They Work:** Specifically designed to extract juice from citrus fruits like oranges, lemons, and grapefruits, either manually or electrically.

- **Pros:** Simple to use, affordable, and perfect for citrus fruits.
- **Cons:** Limited to citrus fruits and not versatile for other types of produce.

4. Manual Juicers:

- **How They Work**: Operate by hand-cranking or pressing, requiring manual effort to extract juice.

- **Pros:** Affordable, portable, and quiet; good for small quantities and specific types of produce like wheatgrass.
- **Cons:** Labor-intensive, slower, and typically less efficient for large quantities.

Essential Juicing Equipment

In addition to a juicer, having the following equipment can enhance your juicing experience:

- **Cutting Board and Knife:** For chopping fruits and vegetables into pieces that fit into your juicer.

- **Strainer or Cheesecloth:** To remove any remaining pulp if you prefer a smoother juice.

- **Storage Containers:** Glass jars or bottles with airtight lids to store juice and maintain freshness.

- **Brush or Scrubber:** For cleaning produce thoroughly before juicing.

Choosing the Right Ingredients

Selecting high-quality ingredients is crucial for getting the best out of your juices:

- **Freshness:** Use fresh, organic fruits and vegetables whenever possible to maximize nutrient content and avoid pesticides.

- **Variety:** Incorporate a wide range of fruits and vegetables to ensure a diverse nutrient intake.

- **Balance:** Combine fruits and vegetables in a way that balances flavors and nutritional benefits. For example, mixing sweet fruits with leafy greens can create a more palatable and nutrient-rich juice.

- **Seasonal Produce**: Opt for seasonal produce to ensure the freshest and most nutrient-dense ingredients.

By understanding these basics, you'll be well-equipped to start your juicing journey and enjoy all the benefits it has to offer. In the following chapters, we'll delve deeper into the nutritional aspects, provide practical juicing tips, and offer a variety of delicious recipes to support your weight loss and health goals.

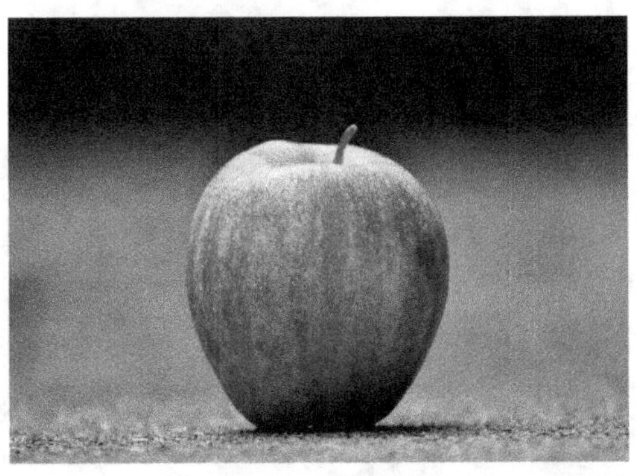

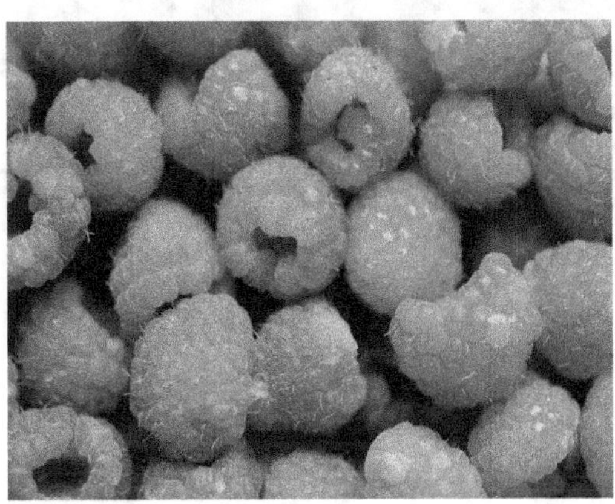

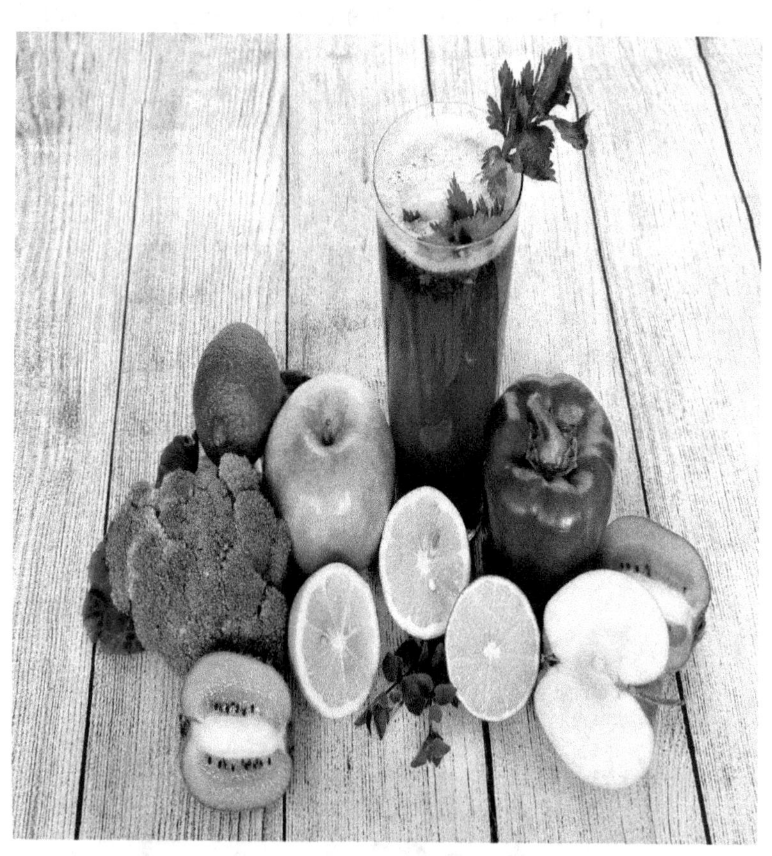

CHAPTER TWO

Nutritional Benefits of Juicing

Vitamins and Minerals

Juicing allows you to access a broad spectrum of essential vitamins and minerals that are crucial for maintaining optimal health:

- **Vitamin A:** Found in carrots, sweet potatoes, and leafy greens, vitamin A supports eye health, immune function, and skin health.

- **Vitamin C:** Present in citrus fruits, strawberries, and bell peppers, vitamin C boosts the immune system, promotes collagen production, and acts as a powerful antioxidant.

- **Vitamin K:** Abundant in kale, spinach, and broccoli, vitamin K is essential for blood clotting and bone health.

- **Potassium:** Bananas, oranges, and tomatoes are rich in potassium, which helps regulate blood pressure, fluid balance, and muscle function.

- **Folate:** Spinach, beets, and avocados provide folate, important for DNA synthesis and repair, and crucial during pregnancy.

Antioxidants and Phytochemicals

Juicing concentrates antioxidants and phytochemicals, which have numerous health benefits:

- **Antioxidants**: Compounds like vitamin C, vitamin E, and beta-carotene neutralize free radicals, reducing oxidative stress and lowering the risk of chronic diseases such as heart disease and cancer.

- **Phytochemicals:** Found in a variety of plant foods, these compounds have anti-inflammatory, anti-cancer, and immune-boosting properties. Examples include flavonoids in berries, lycopene in tomatoes, and sulforaphane in cruciferous vegetables.

Fiber and Digestion

While traditional juicing removes most of the fiber from fruits and vegetables, you can still benefit from soluble fiber and digestive enzymes:

- **Soluble Fiber**: Some soluble fiber remains in the juice, which can help regulate blood sugar levels and support heart health.

- **Digestive Enzymes**: Fresh juices contain natural enzymes that aid digestion and improve nutrient absorption, promoting a healthy digestive system.

Hydration and Detoxification

Juicing provides an excellent way to stay hydrated and support the body's natural detoxification processes:

- **Hydration:** The high water content in fresh juices helps maintain proper hydration, essential for overall health and optimal body function.

- **Detoxification**: Ingredients like cucumber, celery, and lemon support the liver and kidneys in detoxifying the body, flushing out toxins, and improving overall health.

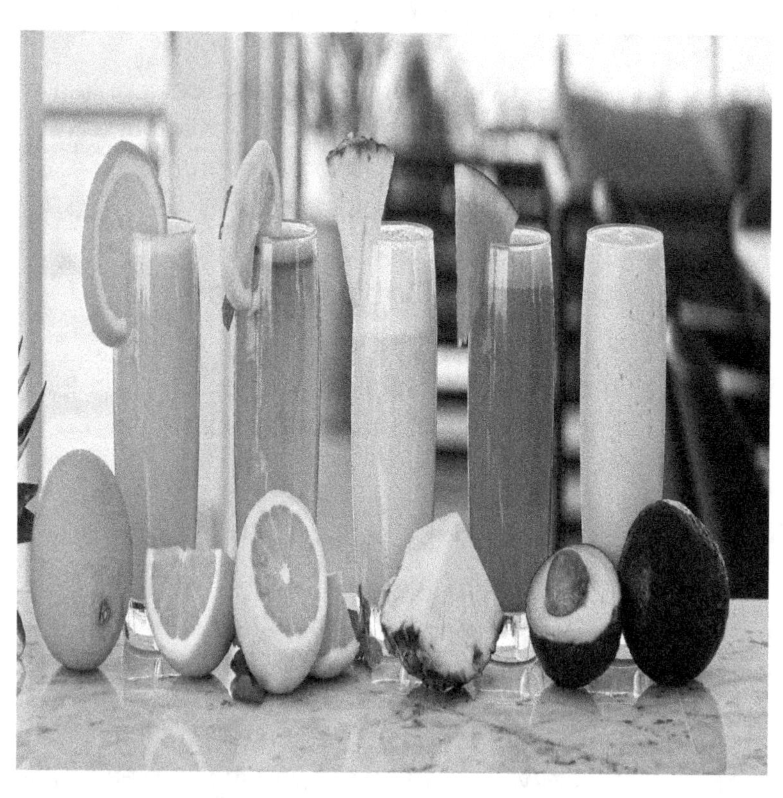

CHAPTER THREE

Preparing for a Juice Diet

Embarking on a juice diet requires careful preparation to ensure success and maximize the benefits. This chapter will guide you through setting realistic goals, planning your juicing schedule, shopping for fresh produce, and making necessary pre-juicing preparations. With the right approach, you can create a sustainable and effective juice diet that supports your weight loss and health goals.

Setting Realistic Goals

Before starting your juice diet, it's important to establish clear and achievable goals:

1. **Define Your Objectives:**

   - Determine what you want to achieve with your juice diet, such as weight loss, detoxification, increased energy, or improved nutrient intake.
   - Set specific, measurable, and time-bound goals to track your progress effectively.

2. **Assess Your Starting Point:**

- Evaluate your current diet, lifestyle, and health status to understand where you're starting from.

- Consider consulting a healthcare professional, especially if you have any underlying health conditions.

3. **Create a Plan:**

- Outline a plan that includes the duration of your juice diet, the types of juices you'll consume, and how you'll incorporate them into your daily routine.

- Set short-term and long-term milestones to keep you motivated and focused.

Planning Your Juicing Schedule

A well-structured juicing schedule is key to maintaining consistency and achieving your goals:

1. **Daily Juicing Routine:**

- Decide how many juices you'll consume each day and at what times (e.g., breakfast, mid-morning, lunch, afternoon, and dinner).

- Aim to include a variety of juices to ensure a balanced intake of nutrients.

2. Meal Replacement:

- Determine which meals or snacks you'll replace with juice. For example, you might replace breakfast and lunch with juice and have a light, healthy dinner.

- Ensure that your juice meals provide adequate calories and nutrients to sustain your energy levels.

3. Juicing Frequency:

- Decide whether you'll juice daily or incorporate juice-only days into your week. Some people find success with a mix of juicing days and regular eating days.

Shopping for Fresh Produce

Selecting high-quality ingredients is crucial for the success of your juice diet:

1. **Create a Shopping List:**

- List the fruits and vegetables you'll need for your juice recipes. Include a variety of colors and types to ensure a diverse nutrient profile.

- Add any additional ingredients like herbs, spices, and superfoods.

2. **Choose Organic:**

- Whenever possible, opt for organic produce to avoid pesticides and chemicals.

- Prioritize buying organic for produce with thin skins or those known to have higher pesticide residues (e.g., apples, berries, spinach).

3. **Buy Fresh and Seasonal:**

- Select fresh, ripe produce for the best flavor and nutrient content.

- Buying seasonal produce can enhance the taste and nutritional value of your juices while often being more cost-effective.

4. **Storage Tips:**

- Store your produce properly to maintain freshness. Keep leafy greens and herbs in the refrigerator and store fruits in a cool, dry place.

- Use breathable bags or containers to extend the shelf life of your produce.

Pre-Juicing Preparations

Proper preparation can streamline your juicing process and ensure you get the most out of your ingredients:

1. **Wash and Prep Produce:**

- Wash all fruits and vegetables thoroughly to remove dirt and pesticides. Use a produce wash or a mixture of vinegar and water for added cleaning.

- Peel, core, and chop produce as needed to fit into your juicer. Removing seeds and tough skins can improve the texture and flavor of your juice.

2. **Batch Prep:**

- Consider preparing your ingredients in batches to save time. Pre-chop and store them in airtight containers in the refrigerator for up to a few days.

- Label containers with the date to keep track of freshness.

3. **Juicing Setup:**

- Set up your juicing station with all necessary equipment, including your juicer, cutting board, knife, and storage containers.

- Ensure your juicer is clean and in good working condition before you start.

4. **Plan for Clean-Up:**

- Juicing can be messy, so plan for clean-up. Line your juicer's pulp bin with a compostable bag for easy disposal, and have a cleaning brush and soapy water ready for quick cleaning.

By setting realistic goals, planning a structured juicing schedule, shopping wisely for fresh produce, and preparing efficiently, you'll set yourself up for a successful juice diet.

CHAPTER FOUR

Juicing Recipes for Weight Loss

These recipes incorporate a variety of fruits, vegetables, and other beneficial ingredients to help you stay full, energized, and on track with your health journey. Each recipe includes a brief description, the ingredients needed, and easy-to-follow instructions.

Green Detox Juice

This juice is packed with leafy greens and detoxifying ingredients to help cleanse your body and boost your metabolism.

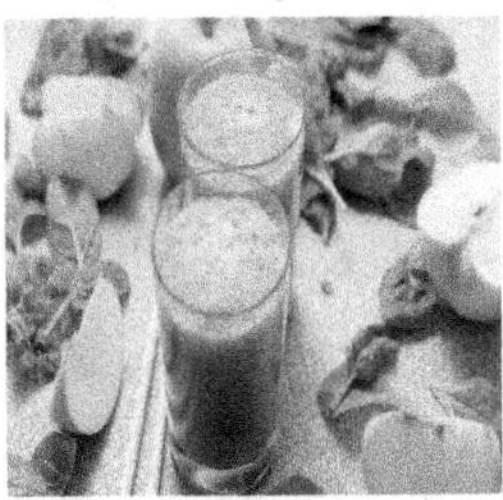

Ingredients:

- 1 cucumber
- 1 green apple
- 1 cup spinach
- 1 lemon (juiced)
- 1-inch piece of ginger

- 1 celery stalk
- 1/2 cup water (optional for consistency)

Instructions:

1. Wash all the ingredients thoroughly.

2. Cut the cucumber, apple, and celery into pieces that fit into your juicer or blender.

3. If using a blender, blend all the ingredients until smooth. If the juice is too thick, add a little water.

4. If preferred, separate the pulp from the juice by straining it through cheesecloth or a fine mesh sieve.

5. Transfer the juice to a glass and squeeze in the lemon juice.

6. Stir well and enjoy immediately for maximum freshness and nutrient content.

Tropical Fat Burner

This sweet and tangy juice combines tropical fruits with metabolism-boosting ingredients to help burn fat.

Ingredients:

- 1 cup pineapple chunks
- 1 orange, peeled
- 1 carrot
- 1/2 lime, peeled
- 1-inch piece of turmeric
- 1/2 teaspoon cayenne pepper (optional, for an extra metabolism boost)

Instructions:

1. Wash all the ingredients.

2. Chop the pineapple, carrot, and turmeric into pieces.

3. Juice the pineapple, orange, carrot, lime, and turmeric.
4. Stir in the cayenne pepper, if using, and mix well before drinking.

Berry Blast Juice

This antioxidant-rich juice helps fight inflammation and supports overall health while aiding in weight loss.

Ingredients:

- 1 cup strawberries

- 1/2 cup blueberries
- 1/2 cup raspberries
- 1 apple
- 1 handful of spinach
- 1/2 lemon, peeled

Instructions:

1. Wash all the berries, apples, and spinach.

2. Cut the apple into pieces.

3. Juice the strawberries, blueberries, raspberries, apple, spinach, and lemon.

4. Stir the juice and enjoy immediately

Refreshing Cucumber Mint Juice

This hydrating juice is perfect for hot days and helps keep you feeling full and refreshed.

Ingredients:

- 1 cucumber
- 1 green apple
- 1/2 lemon, peeled
- 5-6 fresh mint leaves
- 1 cup water (optional, for a lighter juice)

Instructions:

1. Wash all the ingredients.

2. Chop the cucumber and apple into pieces.

3. Juice the cucumber, apple, lemon, and mint leaves.

4. Add water if desired, stir well, and serve chilled.

Spicy Green Lemonade

This tangy and spicy juice combines citrus with green vegetables and a hint of heat to kickstart your metabolism.

Ingredients:

- 1 green apple
- 1 cucumber
- 1 handful of kale
- 1/2 lemon, peeled
- 1-inch piece of ginger
- 1/2 jalapeño pepper (optional, for spice)

Instructions:

1. Wash all the ingredients.

2. Chop the apple, cucumber, ginger, and jalapeño into pieces.

3. Juice the apple, cucumber, kale, lemon, ginger, and jalapeño.

4. Mix well and serve immediately.

Beetroot Power Juice

This juice is rich in antioxidants and nitrates, supporting blood flow and stamina, which can enhance weight loss efforts.

Ingredients:

- 1 beetroot
- 2 carrots
- 1 apple
- 1-inch piece of ginger
- 1/2 lemon, peeled

Instructions:

1. Wash all the ingredients.

2. Peel and chop the beetroot, carrots, apple, and ginger into pieces.

3. Juice the beetroot, carrots, apple, ginger, and lemon.

4. Stir the juice and enjoy it fresh.

Green Protein Juice

This juice incorporates protein to help keep you full and support muscle maintenance while losing weight.

Ingredients:

- 1 handful of spinach
- 1 handful of kale
- 1 cucumber
- 1 green apple
- 1/2 lemon, peeled
- 1 tablespoon of chia seeds, steeped for ten minutes in water

Instructions:

1. Wash all the ingredients.

2. Chop the cucumber and apple into pieces.

3. Juice the spinach, kale, cucumber, apple, and lemon.

4. Stir in the soaked chia seeds and mix well before drinking.

Citrus and Carrot Juice

This bright and refreshing juice is packed with vitamin C and beta-carotene, helping to boost your immune system and support healthy skin.

Ingredients:

- 2 oranges, peeled
- 2 carrots
- 1/2 grapefruit, peeled
- 1-inch piece of turmeric
- 1/2 lemon, peeled

Instructions:

1. Wash all the ingredients.

2. Peel and chop the oranges, carrots, grapefruit, turmeric, and lemon.

3. Juice all the ingredients together.

4. Stir the juice well and enjoy.

Apple and Celery Cleanser

This simple yet effective juice helps cleanse your body and reduce bloating, supporting your weight loss efforts.

Ingredients:

- 2 green apples
- 3 celery stalks
- 1/2 cucumber
- 1/2 lemon, peeled
- 1 handful of parsley

Instructions:

1. Wash all the ingredients.

2. Chop the apples, celery, cucumber, and lemon into pieces.

3. Juice the apples, celery, cucumber, lemon, and parsley

4. .Mix the juice and serve immediately.

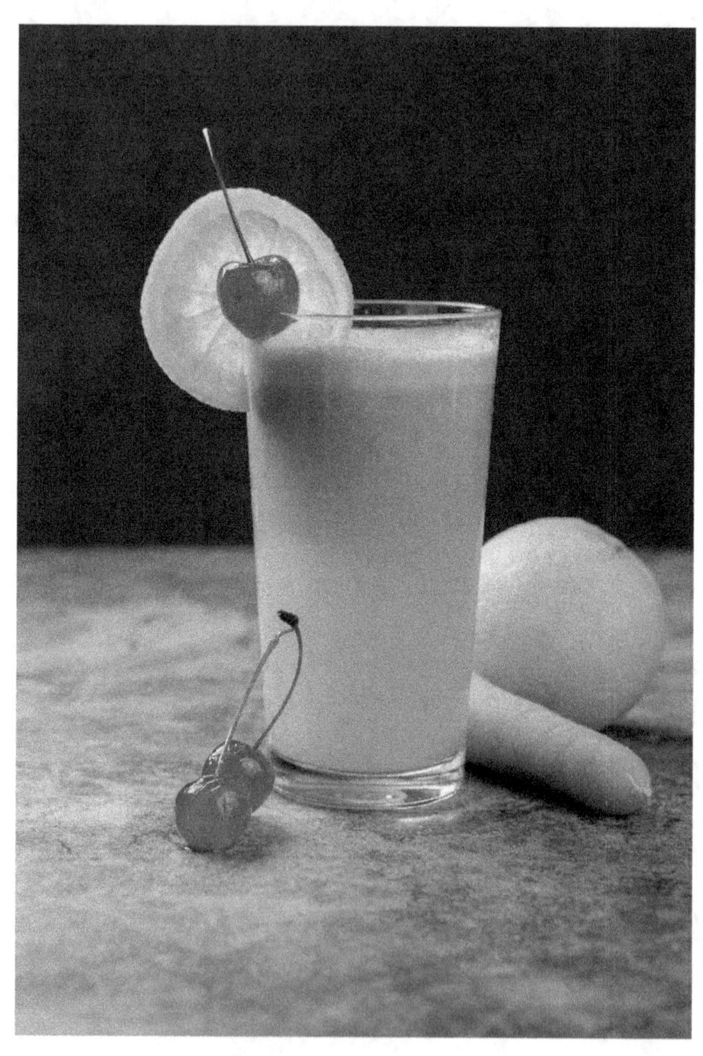

CHAPTER FIVE

Incorporating Juicing into Your Daily Routine

Integrating juicing into your daily life can significantly enhance your health and support your weight loss goals. This chapter provides practical tips on how to seamlessly include juices in your diet, whether as meal replacements, snacks, or complementary additions to your meals.

Morning Boost: Juicing for Breakfast

Starting your day with a nutrient-dense juice can energize you and set a positive tone for the rest of the day:

1. **Wake-Up Hydration:**

- Drink a glass of water or warm lemon water first thing in the morning to hydrate and kickstart your metabolism.

- Follow with a fresh juice rich in vitamins and minerals, such as the Green Detox Juice or

Citrus and Carrot Juice, to fuel your body with essential nutrients.

2. Meal Replacement:

- If you prefer a light breakfast or are on a juice cleanse, replace your morning meal with a juice that includes both fruits and vegetables for balanced nutrition.

- Add a tablespoon of chia seeds or a scoop of protein powder to your juice to keep you fuller for longer and provide additional nutrients.

Mid-Morning Snack: Staying Energized

A mid-morning juice can help maintain your energy levels and prevent unhealthy snacking:

1. Portable Options:

- Prepare your juice in the morning and store it in an airtight container or a thermos to keep it fresh and take it with you to work or on-the-go.

- Opt for juices that are high in fiber and low in sugar, such as the Apple and Celery Cleanser, to avoid energy crashes.

2. **Combining with Snacks:**

- Pair your juice with a handful of nuts, a piece of whole fruit, or a small serving of yogurt to create a balanced, satisfying snack.

- This mixture can provide you long-lasting energy and help balance your blood sugar levels.

Lunchtime: Enhancing or Replacing Meals

Incorporating juice into your lunch can either complement your meal or serve as a meal replacement:

1. **Complementary Juices:**

- Pair your regular lunch with a nutrient-rich juice to boost your intake of vitamins and minerals.

- For example, enjoy the Beetroot Power Juice alongside a salad or a whole grain wrap.

2. **Meal Replacement:**

- On days when you prefer a lighter meal or are following a juice cleanse, replace lunch with a filling juice like the Green Protein Juice.

- Ensure the juice includes a mix of vegetables, fruits, and protein to provide balanced nutrition.

Afternoon Pick-Me-Up: Beating the Slump

Combat the afternoon energy slump with a revitalizing juice:

1. **Refreshing Options:**

- Choose hydrating and invigorating juices such as the Refreshing Cucumber Mint Juice to rehydrate and refresh yourself.

- Adding ingredients like ginger or cayenne pepper can provide a natural energy boost without the need for caffeine.

2. **Snack Substitution:**

- Replace unhealthy snacks like chips or cookies with a nutrient-dense juice to satisfy cravings and keep you on track with your weight loss goals.

- A Berry Blast Juice can be a delicious and antioxidant-rich alternative to sugary snacks.

Evening: Light Dinner or Pre-Dinner Juice

Incorporating juice into your evening routine can help you wind down and prepare for a restful night:

1. **Pre-Dinner Juice:**

- Have a small juice before dinner to curb your appetite and ensure you consume fewer calories during your main meal.

- A Spicy Green Lemonade can stimulate digestion and prepare your stomach for dinner.

2. **Light Dinner Replacement:**

- On lighter eating days or during a cleanse, replace dinner with a filling juice like the Tropical Fat Burner.

- Make sure your juice is rich in nutrients to support your body's overnight repair and recovery processes.

Tips for Successful Daily Juicing

Here are some additional tips to help you integrate juicing into your daily routine effectively:

1. **Consistency is Key:**

   - Aim to include at least one juice in your diet every day to consistently benefit from the nutrients and support your weight loss efforts.

   - Establish a juicing routine that fits your lifestyle and schedule to make it a sustainable habit.

2. **Prep Ahead:**

   - Prepare your ingredients in advance to save time. Wash, chop, and store them in the fridge, so they're ready to juice when you need them.

   - Consider making large batches of juice and storing them in airtight containers for up to 48 hours, although fresh juice is always best.

3. **Stay Hydrated:**

- Drink plenty of water throughout the day, especially when consuming juices, to stay hydrated and support your body's detoxification processes.

4. **Listen to Your Body:**

- After you start juicing, observe how your body reacts. Adjust your juice ingredients and timing based on your energy levels, hunger cues, and digestive comfort.

- If you feel fatigued or experience digestive discomfort, tweak your juice recipes or frequency.

5. **Balance with Whole Foods:**

- While juicing provides concentrated nutrients, it's important to maintain a balanced diet that includes whole fruits and vegetables, lean proteins, healthy fats, and whole grains.

- Use juicing as a supplement to, not a replacement for, a varied and nutritious diet.

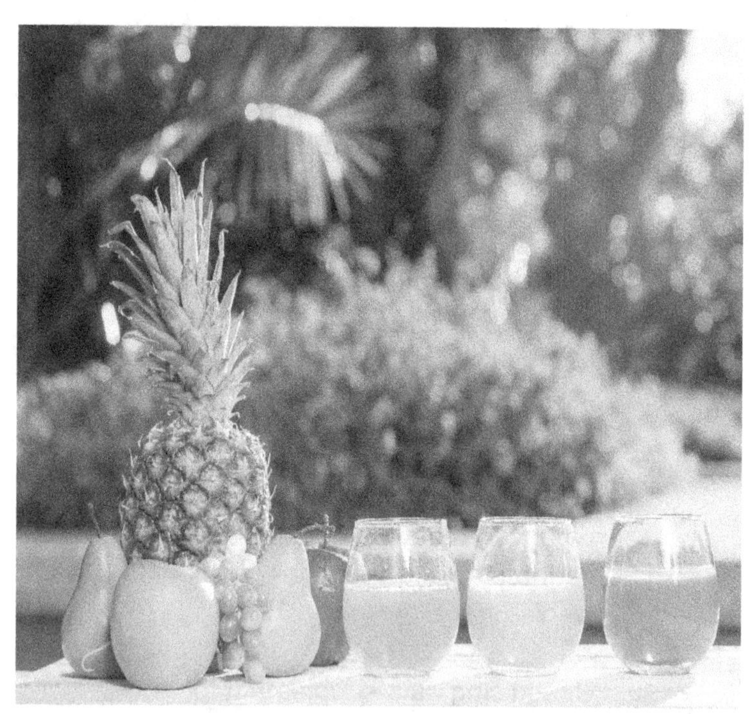

CHAPTER SIX

Tips and Tricks for Successful Juicing

Selecting the best ingredients is crucial for creating delicious and nutritious juices:

1. **Prioritize Freshness:**

- Use fresh, ripe fruits and vegetables for the best taste and maximum nutrient content.

- Avoid produce that is overripe or past its prime, as it can negatively affect the flavor and quality of your juice.

2. **Opt for Organic:**

- Whenever possible, choose organic produce to minimize exposure to pesticides and other chemicals.

- If organic options are not available, thoroughly wash and peel conventional produce to reduce pesticide residues.

3. **Balance Flavors:**

- Combine sweet, tart, and bitter ingredients to create balanced and enjoyable flavors.

- For example, mix sweet fruits like apples and oranges with leafy greens like spinach and kale to create a well-rounded juice.

4. **Incorporate a Variety:**

- Use a diverse range of fruits and vegetables to ensure a broad spectrum of nutrients and prevent flavor fatigue.

- Rotate your ingredients regularly to keep your juices exciting and nutritionally balanced.

Juicing Techniques

Mastering a few essential techniques can enhance your juicing experience:

1. **Prep Your Ingredients:**

- Wash all produce thoroughly to remove dirt and contaminants.

- Peel and core fruits and vegetables as needed, especially if they have tough skins or seeds.

- Chop ingredients into sizes that fit easily into your juicer.

2. **Layering Ingredients:**

- Alternate soft and hard ingredients when feeding them into the juicer to help the machine process everything smoothly.

- Start with high-water content items like cucumbers and finish with leafy greens to maximize juice extraction.

3. **Strain Your Juice:**

- If you prefer a smoother juice, strain it through a fine mesh sieve or cheesecloth to remove any remaining pulp.

- For extra fiber, leave some pulp in your juice or add it to other recipes like soups or smoothies.

4. **Mix and Match:**

- Experiment with different combinations to find your favorite flavors and nutrient profiles.

- Keep a journal of your juice recipes and adjustments to track what works best for you.

Storing Juice

Proper storage techniques can help maintain the quality and freshness of your juice:

1. **Use Airtight Containers:**

- Store juice in airtight glass jars or bottles to minimize oxidation and preserve nutrients.

- Fill containers to the top to reduce air exposure and prolong freshness.

2. **Refrigerate Promptly:**

- Store juice in the refrigerator immediately after juicing to keep it fresh.

- Consume stored juice within 24-48 hours for optimal taste and nutritional value.

3. **Freeze for Later:**

- If you need to store juice for longer periods, consider freezing it in portions.

- Make sure your containers are freezer-safe and allow for some expansion.Thaw in the refrigerator before drinking.

Cleaning Your Juicer

Keeping your juicer clean is essential for hygiene and performance:

1. **Clean Immediately:**

- Clean your juicer right after use to prevent residue from drying and becoming difficult to remove.

- Disassemble the parts and rinse them under warm water.

2. **Use a Brush:**

- Use a small brush to clean the juicer's mesh strainer and other hard-to-reach areas.

- Many juicers come with a cleaning brush specifically designed for this purpose.

3. **Soak in Soapy Water:**

Soak removable parts in warm, soapy water for a few minutes to loosen any stubborn residue.

- Rinse well, then let everything air dry before putting it all back together.

4. **Regular Deep Cleaning:**

- Perform a deep cleaning of your juicer every week or as needed, especially if you juice frequently.

- Check the manufacturer's instructions for specific cleaning recommendations.

Cost-Saving Tips

Juicing can be economical with a few savvy strategies:

1. **Buy in Bulk:**

- Purchase fruits and vegetables in bulk to save money, especially when they are in season.

- Join a local CSA (Community Supported Agriculture) program or shop at farmers' markets for fresh, affordable produce.

2. **Use Seasonal Produce:**

- Choose seasonal fruits and vegetables to benefit from lower prices and better quality.

- Plan your juice recipes around what is in season to keep costs down.

3. **Grow Your Own:**

- Consider growing your own herbs, greens, and small fruits if you have the space and time.

- Homegrown produce can be a cost-effective and rewarding addition to your juicing routine.

4. **Minimize Waste:**

- Use the pulp from juicing in other recipes, such as soups, muffins, or composting for your garden.

- Store and preserve excess produce by freezing or canning to extend its shelf life.

Listening to Your Body

Pay attention to how your body responds to juicing:

1. **Start Gradually:**

- If you're new to juicing, start with one juice a day and gradually increase as your body adjusts.

- Observe how different ingredients affect you and adjust accordingly.

2. **Monitor Your Energy Levels:**

- Note any changes in your energy levels, digestion, and overall well-being.

- Adjust the timing and composition of your juices to best support your body's needs.

3. **Stay Hydrated:**

- Drink plenty of water alongside your juices to stay hydrated and support your body's detoxification processes.

- Avoid relying solely on juice for hydration.

4. **Balance Your Diet:**

- Ensure that juicing complements a balanced diet that includes whole foods, lean proteins, healthy fats, and whole grains.

- Use juicing as a supplement to enhance your overall nutritional intake.

CHAPTER SEVEN

Exercise and Juicing for Optimal Results

Combining a juicing regimen with regular exercise can significantly enhance your weight loss efforts and overall health.

The Benefits of Combining Exercise and Juicing

1. **Enhanced Weight Loss:**

- Exercise helps burn calories, build muscle, and boost metabolism, complementing the calorie deficit created by a juice diet.

- Juicing provides essential nutrients that fuel your workouts and aid in recovery.

2. **Improved Energy Levels:**

- Regular physical activity increases your energy levels and stamina, making it easier to stay active throughout the day.

- Nutrient-dense juices can provide a quick energy boost before or after workouts.

3. Detoxification and Recovery:

- Sweating is encouraged by exercise, which aids in the body's detoxification.

- Juicing provides antioxidants and anti-inflammatory compounds that support muscle recovery and reduce post-exercise soreness.

4. Balanced Nutrition:

- Juicing ensures you get a concentrated dose of vitamins, minerals,and phytonutrients to support overall health.

- When combined with a balanced exercise routine, juicing can help maintain nutrient levels and prevent deficiencies.

Selecting the Right Types of Exercises

1. Cardiovascular Exercise:

- Activities such as running, cycling, swimming, and dancing are excellent for burning calories and improving heart health.

- Aim for 150 minutes or 75 minutes of high-intensity or moderate- intensity cardio per week at minimum.

2. Strength Training:

- Incorporate weight lifting, resistance band exercises, or bodyweight workouts to build muscle and boost metabolism.

- Aim for two or three sessions of strength training every week, paying particular attention to the main muscle groups.

3. Flexibility and Balance:

- Activities like yoga, Pilates, and stretching improve flexibility, balance, and overall well-being.

- Include flexibility and balance exercises in your routine two to three times per week.

4. High-Intensity Interval Training (HIIT):

- HIIT involves short bursts of intense exercise followed by brief rest periods, which can be highly effective for burning fat and improving fitness.

- Aim for one to two HIIT sessions per week, ensuring proper form and adequate rest.

Timing Your Workouts and Juicing

1. **Pre-Workout Juices:**

- Consume a juice 30-60 minutes before exercise to provide quick-digesting carbohydrates and energy.

- Ideal pre-workout juices include ingredients like apples, oranges, beets, and carrots.

Pre-Workout Juice Recipe:

- ➢ **Energizing Beet Juice:**

- 1 beetroot
- 1 apple
- 1 carrot
- 1/2 lemon, peeled
- 1-inch piece of ginger

Instructions:

- Wash and chop the ingredients.

- Juice all the ingredients and stir well.

- Drink 30 minutes before your workout.

2. **Post-Workout Juices:**

- Consume a juice within 30 minutes after exercise to replenish glycogen stores, hydrate, and provide essential nutrients for recovery.

- Ideal post-workout juices include ingredients like leafy greens, citrus fruits, and protein-rich add-ins like chia seeds.

Post-Workout Juice Recipe:

➤ **Recovery Green Juice:**

- 1 cucumber
- 2 celery stalks
- 1 handful of spinach
- 1 apple
- 1/2 lemon, peeled
- 1 tablespoon of chia seeds, steeped for ten minutes in water.

Instructions:

- Wash and chop the ingredients.

- Juice all the ingredients except chia seeds.

- Stir in soaked chia seeds and drink immediately after your workout.

Hydration and Juicing:

- Stay hydrated throughout the day by drinking water and incorporating hydrating juices.

- Avoid relying solely on juices for hydration, as water is essential for optimal bodily functions.

Hydrating Juice Recipe:

➢ **Cucumber Mint Hydrator:**

- 1 cucumber
- 1 green apple
- 1/2 lemon, peeled
- 5-6 fresh mint leaves

Instructions:

- Wash and chop the ingredients.

- Juice all the ingredients and stir well.

- Drink throughout the day to stay hydrated.

Creating a Balanced Exercise and Juicing Plan

Set Clear Goals:

- Define your fitness and weight loss goals to tailor your exercise and juicing plan accordingly.

- Establish SMART goals—specific, measurable, achievable, relevant, and time-bound.

Develop a Routine:

- Create a weekly exercise schedule that includes a mix of cardio, strength training, flexibility, and balance exercises.

- Plan your juicing schedule around your workouts to ensure proper nutrient timing.

Listen to Your Body:

- Pay attention to your body's signals and adjust your exercise intensity and juice intake as needed.

- To avoid injury and burnout, make sure you get enough sleep and recuperation.

Monitor Progress:

- Track your workouts, juice recipes, and progress towards your goals in a journal or fitness app.

- Adapt your strategy to your progress and any obstacles you face.

By integrating juicing with a balanced exercise routine, you can maximize your weight loss results and improve your overall health.

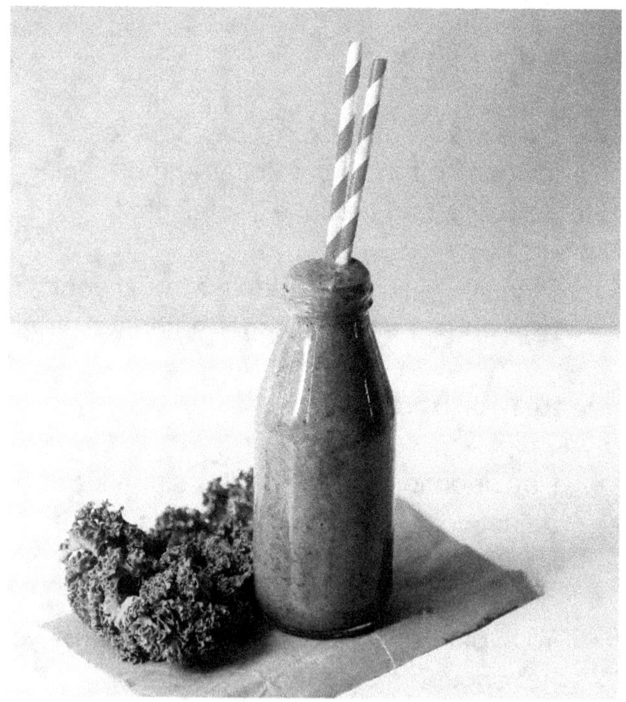

CHAPTER EIGHT

Long-Term Weight Management with Juicing

Maintaining weight loss and achieving long-term health goals requires sustainable habits and lifestyle changes. Juicing can play a crucial role in long-term weight management when integrated thoughtfully into your routine.

Establishing Sustainable Habits

1. **Consistency Over Perfection:**

- Aim for consistency in your juicing and dietary habits rather than striving for perfection.

- Make juicing a regular part of your routine, but don't stress over occasional deviations.

2. **Balanced Nutrition:**

- Enhance your diet with whole foods and juicing to achieve a well-balanced diet.

- Ensure your diet includes a variety of fruits, vegetables, lean proteins, healthy fats, and whole grains.

3. **Mindful Eating:**

- By observing your body's signals of hunger and fullness, cultivate mindful eating.

- Use juices as a way to nourish your body and complement your meals, not as a replacement for mindful eating practices.

4. **Regular Physical Activity:**

- Maintain a consistent exercise routine that includes a mix of cardiovascular, strength training, flexibility, and balance exercises.

- Use juicing to support your energy levels and recovery from workouts.

Incorporating Juicing into Daily Life

1. **Meal Planning and Preparation:**

- Plan your meals and juices ahead of time to ensure you have the necessary ingredients and to avoid last-minute unhealthy choices.

- Batch prepares juices and stores them in airtight containers for convenience.

2. **Balanced Juicing:**

- Focus on juices that combine fruits, vegetables, and other nutrient-dense ingredients to provide a balanced mix of vitamins, minerals, and fiber.

- Avoid juices that are too high in sugar by emphasizing vegetables and low-sugar fruits.

3. **Seasonal and Local Produce:**

- Incorporate seasonal and locally-sourced produce in your juices to enjoy a variety of flavors and nutrients.

- Seasonal produce is often fresher, more nutritious, and more cost-effective.

Monitoring and Adjusting Your Approach

1. **Track Your Progress:**

- Keep a journal or use an app to track your juicing habits, dietary intake, exercise routine, and progress toward your weight management goals.

- Review your entries regularly to identify patterns, successes, and areas for improvement.

2. **Listen to Your Body:**

- Pay attention to how your body responds to different juices and dietary changes.

- Adjust your juicing recipes and frequency based on your energy levels, digestion, and overall well-being.

3. **Set Realistic Goals:**

- Establish achievable long-term goals for weight management and health, such as maintaining a certain weight range, improving fitness levels, or achieving specific health milestones.

- Break these goals into smaller, manageable steps to stay motivated and on track.

4. **Stay Flexible:**

- Be flexible and adaptable with your juicing and dietary habits. Life circumstances and individual needs change over time, and your approach should reflect that.

- Allow for occasional indulgences and variations without feeling guilty.

Overcoming Common Challenges

1. **Plateaus:**

- Weight loss plateaus are common. If you hit a plateau, reassess your diet and exercise routine to identify areas for improvement.

- Consider varying your juice recipes, increasing your physical activity, or consulting a nutritionist for personalized advice.

2. **Social and Lifestyle Factors:**

- Social events, travel, and busy schedules can disrupt your juicing routine. Plan ahead by preparing portable juices or choosing healthy options when dining out.

- Communicate your goals to friends and family for support and understanding.

3. **Boredom and Monotony:**

- Prevent boredom by experimenting with new juice recipes and ingredients regularly.

- Join online communities or follow juicing blogs and social media accounts for inspiration and new ideas.

4. **Nutrient Deficiencies:**

- Ensure you are getting a comprehensive range of nutrients by incorporating a variety of whole foods in addition to your juices.

- Consider periodic blood tests to monitor nutrient levels and address any deficiencies with dietary adjustments or supplements.

Maintaining a Positive Mindset

1. **Celebrate Small Wins:**

- No matter how little your development is, acknowledge it and appreciate it.This can boost your motivation and reinforce positive habits.

- Set non-food-related rewards for achieving milestones, such as treating yourself to a new workout outfit or a relaxing spa day.

2. **Stay Informed:**

- Educate yourself about nutrition, fitness, and wellness to make informed decisions about your health.

- Stay updated with new research and trends in juicing and healthy living.

3. **Build a Support System:**

- Surround yourself with supportive friends, family, and community members who encourage your healthy lifestyle.

- Consider joining a weight loss or wellness group for additional support and accountability.

4. **Practice Self-Compassion:**

- Be kind to yourself during your weight management journey. Understand that setbacks are a natural part of the process. Focus on progress rather than perfection, and remind yourself of the positive changes you've made.

- The key is to maintain a balanced, flexible approach that suits your lifestyle and individual needs.

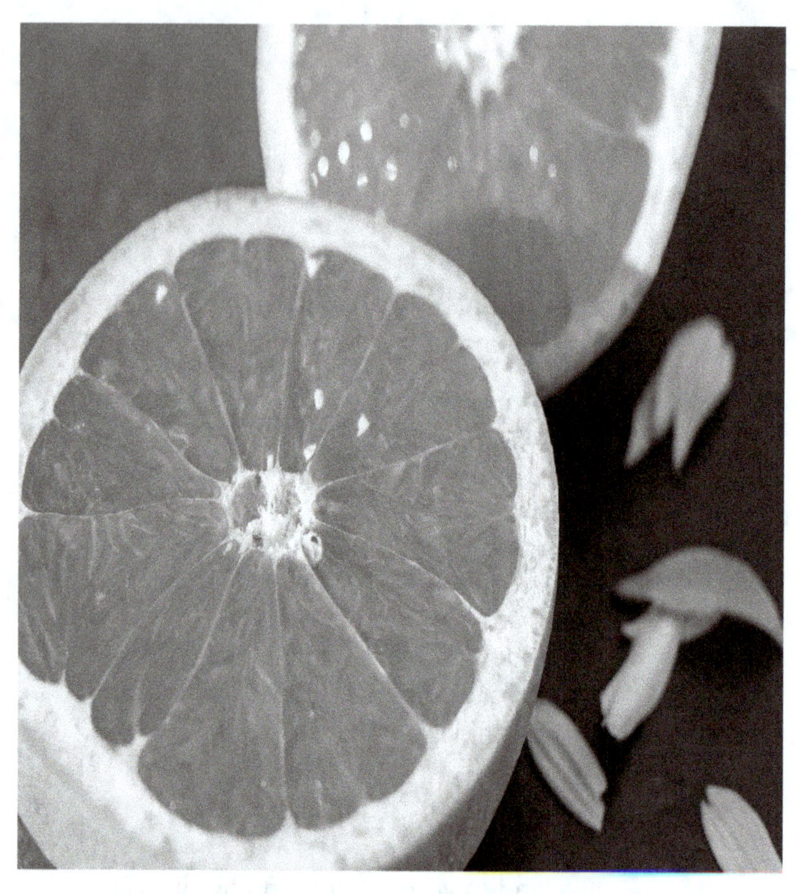

CHAPTER NINE

Frequently Asked Questions

General Juicing Questions

Q1: What is juicing?

A1: Juicing is the process of extracting juice from fruits and vegetables, separating the liquid from the fiber to create a nutrient-dense drink. It allows you to consume a concentrated amount of vitamins, minerals, and phytonutrients in a convenient and delicious form.

Q2: What are the benefits of juicing?

A2: Juicing can provide numerous benefits, including improved digestion, increased nutrient intake, enhanced energy levels, better hydration, and support for weight loss. It can also help detoxify the body and boost the immune system.

Q3: How often should I drink juice?

A3: This depends on your personal health goals and lifestyle. For general health, one juice per day is a good start. For more intensive weight loss or detox goals, you might drink 2-3 juices a day. Always pay attention to your body, and if in doubt, get advice from a medical practitioner.

Q4: Can juicing replace meals?

A4: While juicing can replace meals during short-term cleanses, it's not advisable to rely solely on juice for long-term nutrition. Use juices to supplement a balanced diet that includes whole foods for a
well-rounded nutrient intake.

Q5: Is juicing expensive?

A5: Juicing can be cost-effective if you buy in-season and local produce, purchase in bulk, or grow your own fruits and vegetables. Investing in a good juicer and using budget-friendly ingredients can also help manage costs.

Health and Safety

Q6: Are there any risks associated with juicing?

A6: While juicing is generally safe, there are a few risks to be aware of. An excessive intake of fruit juice can result in a high sugar intake. Additionally, those with specific health conditions, like diabetes or kidney problems, should consult a healthcare professional before starting a juicing regimen.

Q7: Can juicing help with weight loss?

A7: Yes, juicing can aid in weight loss by providing low-calorie, nutrient-dense drinks that can replace higher-calorie meals and snacks. It also helps in reducing cravings and improving overall nutrition. Combining juicing with a balanced diet and regular exercise enhances weight loss efforts.

Q8: What if I have dietary restrictions?

A8: Juicing is versatile and can accommodate various dietary restrictions. You can choose ingredients that align with your dietary needs, such as gluten-free, dairy-free, or low-sugar options. Always check for any food allergies or intolerances before juicing new ingredients.

Q9: How can I avoid nutrient deficiencies while juicing?

A9: Ensure you use a variety of fruits and vegetables to get a broad spectrum of nutrients. Incorporate juices as part of a balanced diet that includes whole foods, lean proteins, healthy fats, and grains. Monitoring nutritional levels can be aided by routine blood testing.

Q10: Is it safe to juice while pregnant or breastfeeding?

A10: Pregnant or breastfeeding women should consult with a healthcare provider before starting a juicing regimen. While fresh juices can provide beneficial nutrients, it's essential to ensure they are part of a balanced diet that meets all nutritional needs during these critical periods.

Practical Tips

Q11: What type of juicer should I use?

A11: The type of juicer depends on your needs and budget. Centrifugal juicers are fast and affordable but may produce less juice and lower nutrient quality. Masticating (slow) juicers are more expensive but extract more juice and retain more nutrients. Consider your priorities when choosing a juicer.

Q12: How do I store fresh juice?

A12: Store fresh juice in airtight glass containers in the refrigerator. Consume within 24-48 hours for optimal freshness and nutrient retention. If you need to store juice for longer, consider freezing it in portions and thawing before drinking.

Q13: Can I juice frozen fruits and vegetables?

A13: Yes, you can juice frozen fruits and vegetables, though fresh produce is generally preferred for optimal taste and nutrient content. Thaw frozen items slightly before juicing to prevent damage to your juicer.

Q14: How do I clean my juicer?

A14: Clean your juicer immediately after use to prevent residue build up. After disassembling the pieces, give them a warm water rinse.Use a brush to clean the mesh strainer and other small areas. Soak parts in soapy water if needed, and allow to air dry before reassembling.

Q15: Can I use the pulp left after juicing?

A15: Yes, the pulp can be used in various recipes to add fiber and nutrients. Consider adding it to soups, stews, muffins, or as compost for your garden. You can also blend it into smoothies for added texture and nutrition.

Personalizing Your Juicing Journey

Q16: How do I create my own juice recipes?

A16: Start by selecting a mix of fruits and vegetables you enjoy. Aim for a balance of flavors by combining sweet, tart, and bitter ingredients. Experiment with different combinations and proportions until you find what you like. Keep track of your recipes and tweak them based on your taste and nutritional needs.

Q17: Can I juice while traveling?

A17: While traveling, you can maintain your juicing habits by bringing portable juicers or purchasing fresh juices from local markets and juice bars. Plan ahead and research places where you can find healthy juice options at your destination.

Q18: What if I don't like the taste of vegetable juices?

A18: Start by mixing vegetables with fruits to balance the taste. For example, add apples, pineapples, or oranges to green juices. Gradually increase the vegetable content as you get used to the flavors. Adding herbs like mint or ginger can also enhance the taste.

Q19: How can I involve my family in juicing?

A19: Involve your family by letting them choose their favorite fruits and vegetables for juicing. Make juicing a fun and educational activity by explaining the health benefits and experimenting with different recipes together. Children often enjoy creating their own juice combinations.

Q20: How do I stay motivated to juice regularly?

A20: Set specific health goals and track your progress to stay motivated. Keep a variety of recipes to prevent boredom and make juicing enjoyable. Join online communities or groups for support and inspiration. Remind yourself of the benefits and positive changes juicing brings to your health.

These frequently asked questions cover a wide range of topics to help you get the most out of your juicing journey.

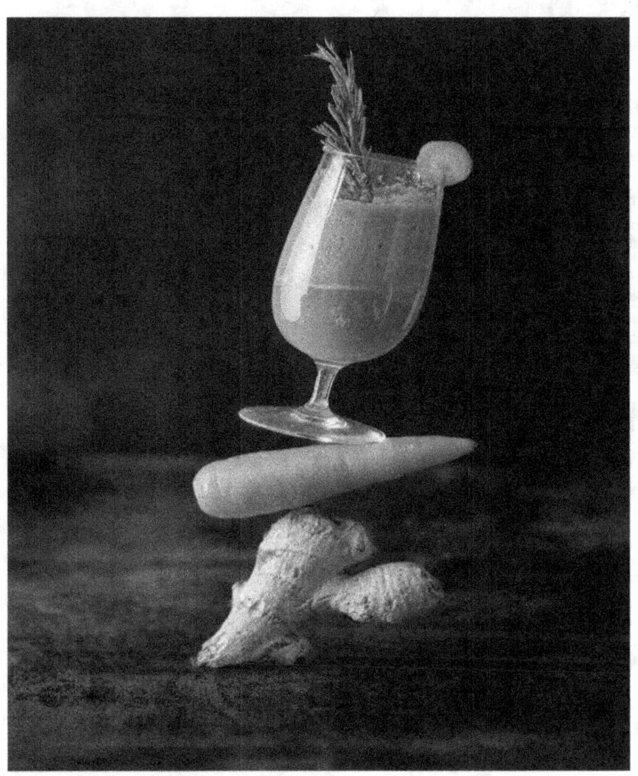

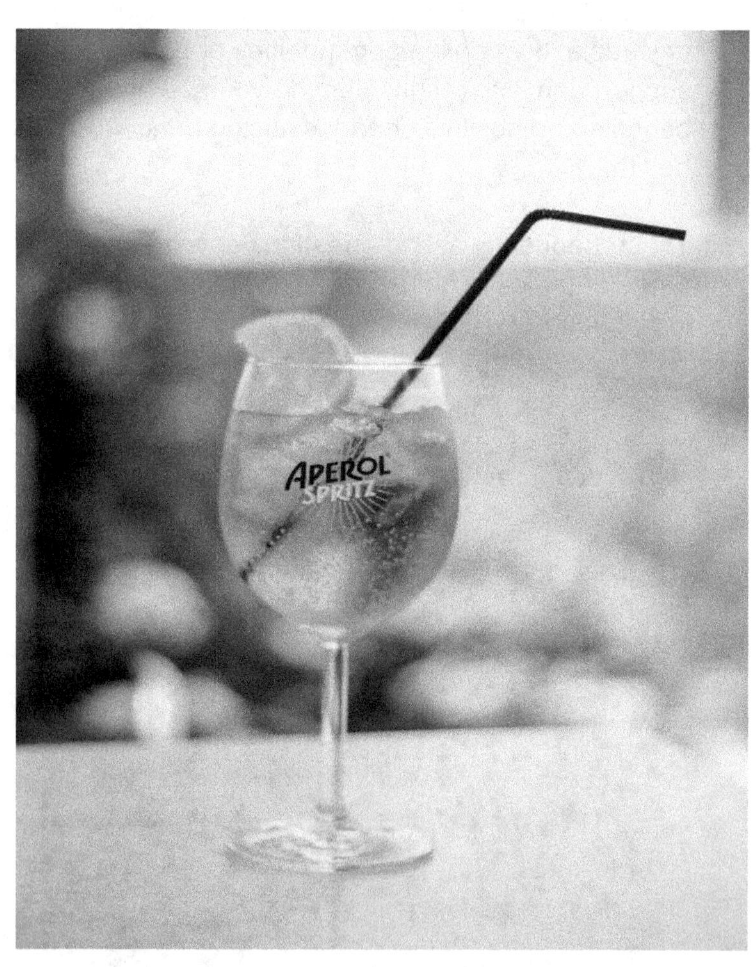
APEROL
SPRITZ

CHAPTER TEN

Moving forward

Stay Informed:

Keep educating yourself about nutrition, fitness, and wellness. The more you know, the better equipped you'll be to make informed decisions about your health.

Seek Support:

Join juicing communities, online forums, or local groups to connect with like-minded individuals. Exchanges of insights and counsel can be immensely inspiring.

Be Flexible:

Adapt your juicing and dietary habits to fit your lifestyle and individual needs. Life is dynamic, and your approach should be too.

Celebrate Progress:

Celebrate and acknowledge all of your accomplishments, no matter how tiny. This maintains your motivation and rewards good behavior.

Listen to Your Body:

Pay attention to how your body responds to different juices and routines. Adjust as needed to ensure you feel your best.

Embarking on a juicing journey for weight loss and overall health is a transformative step towards a healthier, more vibrant life. Throughout this book, we've explored the numerous benefits of juicing, and provided practical guidance.

Final Thoughts

Juicing is more than just a dietary choice; it's a lifestyle change that can significantly enhance your health and well-being. By making juicing a regular part of your routine, you are investing in your long-term health and happiness. Remember to enjoy the process, be patient with yourself, and celebrate each step forward on your journey to a healthier, more vibrant life.

Conclusion

In conclusion, juicing can be a valuable addition to a weight loss regimen when approached with balance and mindfulness. The practice of juicing offers an efficient means of incorporating a variety of nutrient-dense fruits and vegetables into one's diet, providing essential vitamins, minerals, and antioxidants. These elements support overall health, aid in digestion, and promote detoxification, all of which are vital aspects of successful weight loss.

However, it's crucial to recognize that juicing should complement a well-rounded diet and lifestyle that includes regular exercise and healthy eating habits. While juices can be beneficial for weight loss due to their low-calorie content and potential to reduce cravings, they should not replace whole foods entirely. Additionally, being mindful of portion sizes and the sugar content of juices is essential to prevent overconsumption and maintain steady progress towards weight loss goals. By incorporating juicing into a balanced approach to nutrition and fitness, individuals can harness its benefits as a tool for achieving and sustaining a healthier weight.

Bonus

Here's a 7-day daily juice routine specifically designed for weight loss:

Day	Ingredients
Monday	Spinach, cucumber, green apple, lemon, ginger
Tuesday	Carrot, celery, apple, ginger, lemon
Wednesday	Kale, cucumber, celery, green apple, lemon
Thursday	Pineapple, cucumber, mint, lime, spinach
Friday	Beetroot, carrot, cucumber, lemon, ginger
Saturday	Tomato, red bell pepper, celery, parsley, lemon
Sunday	Watermelon, cucumber, mint, lime

Each of these juice blends is designed to be low in calories while providing essential nutrients, promoting hydration, and supporting your weight loss journey.